Cancer Without Fear:

Integrating Complementary and Alternative Medicine with Mainstream Treatment

Julie Moffitt

Printed and bound in the USA
Cover graphics by Bernadette Warman

Printed by Madjulie Music
1521 Cedar Cliff Dr. Suite 203
Camp Hill, PA 17011

This book is dedicated to my husband, Eric Doerfler.
Although the word is not included in the mandala
on the front cover, Love is perhaps the most
powerful healing tool of all.

Introduction

When my friends and family found out I had breast cancer, many of them asked if I was going to write or blog about it. My answer was a resounding "No!" I wasn't ready to announce to the whole world that I had cancer. In fact, I didn't want to talk about it at all. The more I talked about it, the more it would seem real. Plus, many people had already written about dealing with cancer, and I didn't think I had anything new to add to the conversation. If I was going to write, it would just be for my own private journal.

I kept with that line of thinking for quite a few months, even as I weathered my surgeries very well and people were remarking upon how quickly I was bouncing back. It wasn't until I was about halfway through my chemotherapy regimen that I started to rethink my decision. People all around me were amazed at how well I was doing. My husband, a nurse practitioner, and my oncologist were both telling me I was doing better than the average patient. My officemate at work said "If you weren't wearing a turban, I wouldn't even remember that you're doing chemo." I was absolutely certain that my success was due to three things I was doing in addition to my mainstream medical regimen. One, I was using mind-body and holistic therapies: meditation, sound healing therapy, Reiki, and Homeopathy. Two, I was using guided imagery and affirmations to reinforce positive thoughts and to keep my spirits high. Three, I was doing yoga and aerobic exercise regularly. Many cancer patients I talked to weren't utilizing these other options. While I knew there was lots of information available about integrating alternative therapies into treatment, not everyone I had met was aware of it. I finally realized I had a story to tell with a message that could be of use to others.

If you are a cancer patient, I hope that my story in the following pages will be of help to you in getting through your treatments. It certainly made all the difference to me.

The Beginning:
Diagnosis and Choices

Well, at least I won't have to shave my legs for four months!

(My first exclamation when I decided to go ahead with chemotherapy treatment.)

<u>RULE #1</u>
There's a positive side to everything.

When I was first diagnosed with breast cancer, I responded the way I assume most people do: I felt numb. Once the numbness faded I started worrying. When I was growing up, cancer was a devastating diagnosis; it put you in a separate category from everyone else, and was often a death sentence. These days, cancer treatments have improved a great deal, at least for some types of cancer; someone can get a cancer diagnosis and go on to live a happy and healthy life after treatment. Yet the stigma remains. Certain phrases carry a lot of cultural baggage, and "breast cancer" is one of them, especially with all the media attention in the last few years.

So I worried. Perhaps the most upsetting worry was about how and what to tell people. I didn't want them to make a Thing out of it, and I didn't want them to see me differently, just like I didn't want to see *myself* any differently. I almost didn't even want to tell my husband and sister (the two people closest to me) because they would be scared and sad, and I didn't want to inflict that burden on them. I didn't want people to worry about me or feel sorry for me.

I worried that I would miss work if I had to go through a bunch of procedures. I love my job. I am a music teacher, composer and performer, and my work brings me a great deal of joy. My piano students are my musical family, and I didn't want to let them down or miss sharing music with them because of illness. I worried, too, that my finances would suffer if I couldn't work. My husband Eric and I had just built our own house. We had done most of the work ourselves to save money, but we still had considerable debts. We also hadn't sold our previous house, and were paying two mortgages, so financial worries were near the top of my list.

Of course, I worried about what might happen to me and what treatments I would have to go through. Surgery? Reconstruction and perhaps disfigurement? Chemotherapy and the subsequent hair loss and side effects?

Oddly enough, I wasn't really worried that I was going to die, for two reasons. First, at that point my cancer was only classed as Stage One,[1] which made it not too scary; I knew a number of women who had gone through breast cancer treatment at Stage Two and were fine now. Second, I am blessed, or cursed, with the belief that I am invincible and can get through anything. Of course I'm not, but it's a belief I got from my mother, who managed to live a productive and happy life for fifty-one years with multiple sclerosis. She died at 91, still lucid and convinced she'd live another five years. Good role model!

If I was afraid of anything, it was the uncertainly of not knowing what I faced in terms of treatment. Once I had a course of treatment, I could figure out how to deal with it.

I went along in this state of mind for about two weeks, feeling nervous and out of control. Then I thought, *Well, enough of this. Time to be proactive.* I was determined not to let my condition define me, and to face my treatment plans, and subsequent repercussions, on my own terms.

One of the first things I thought about was in what context to see my condition. I have never been comfortable with the metaphors that are so often used in our society when referring to cancer: *battle*, *fight*, *survivor*. It implies that if you

---

[1] Basically stage 1 breast cancer means that the cancer is small and only in the breast tissue or it might be found in lymph nodes close to the breast. More info about cancer staging can be viewed at **http://www.cancerresearchuk.org/about-cancer/breast-cancer/stages-types-grades/number-stages**.

lose the battle, you weren't strong enough. Plus, these are terms which imply cancer is a foreigner swooping in to get you. In fact, the cancer cells were my own cells, horribly, and potentially fatally, out of control. The metaphor that worked for me was to see my goal as bringing my body back into healthy balance.

While our bodies maintain a healthy balance most of the time, for one reason or another (too much stress, adverse genes, etc.), mine had not. I now had a tumor and needed the procedures my doctor was recommending. At the same time, I was aware that **allopathic**[2] (or mainstream) **medicine** wasn't the only thing I could do to help me on my journey to become healthy and cancer-free.

In recent years there has been a great deal of research into **CAM** (the common acronym for Complementary and Alternative Medicine). There are many different kinds within this CAM designation, but some of these are called mind-body therapies. I was fairly familiar with some of the literature on this, plus I had already had some first-hand experience. For one thing, the area of focus in my husband Eric's PhD in Nursing was **psychoneuroimmunology** (PNI), a discipline that studies the continuous interaction of the mind, nervous system, and immune system. Plus, as well as being a Nurse Practitioner, he is also a **classical homeopath**. As you can imagine, holistic and mind-body medicine is a frequent dinner table topic at my house.

I had already spent some time on my own studying **sound healing therapy** and **Reiki.** In fact, it was a goal of mine to become a practitioner of sound healing therapy, but I had dragged my heels. Although I believed it worked, I hadn't made the leap from client to practitioner. I guess I believed and I didn't believe at the same time. In addition to that study, I had meditated and done yoga for years, and had read about and experienced for myself the positive effects of these

---

[2] Terms in bold are in the glossary (Appendix III).

practices. I knew if I integrated some of these modalities into my mainstream health procedures they could have a positive influence on my recovery: the healthier I was in mind and body, the better I would recover from any treatments. These practices, when done regularly, could also help make me a more balanced, spiritually whole person. However, I was going to have to look elsewhere for resources. My cancer treatment center did not integrate these approaches to healing into patient care at all.

You might think I would've gone online to read other people's accounts of their experiences, but I didn't. I didn't want to join a support group or read any blogs. In fact, every time I thought "I should read that literature the Breast Center gave me," I somehow found something else to do. Part of it, no doubt, was because I was in denial. If I joined a group, it would be more real, and I didn't want to think of it as real, at least not in the mainstream medicine sense. I've also never been comfortable in groups; I'm a bit of a loner. The only group I've ever joined was the Lord of the Rings Fan Club, and that was only so I could get the magazines. But the main reason I instinctively shied away from reading about it was that it was depressing. I did not want to spend months and months being unhappy and scared. For one thing, stress has been shown to weaken your immune system, which was the last thing I needed. I wanted to keep living my life as normally as possible, and to fill my mind with positive ideas and thoughts.

I must give some credit to Ann, a colleague of my husband's. She is also a PhD nurse. A few years previously, she had faced much the same thing I was facing, and offered to talk to me about it. I accepted. I didn't know her well, but Eric said that she had used some of the same mind-body techniques that I was contemplating, to great advantage.

Ann encouraged me to go with my gut feeling on this, and that helped me to feel like I was choosing the best approach, because, for all my previous personal experience and my knowledge of the research on the efficacy of mind-body healing and the holistic approach, I knew that some of the people around me would consider this approach crazy new age ideas or pseudo-science nonsense and dismiss it. I was aware that I would be facing some skeptics – particularly my doctors, but also some of my friends and family. Luckily, my husband Eric wasn't among the skeptics. His encouragement and support was a huge factor.

So with Eric and Ann's encouragement, I decided to embark on a joint venture of mainstream medicine plus my own regimen of exercise, meditation, **guided imagery**, and mind-body healing sessions.

<u>BONUS</u>

Although I said earlier that I didn't want to tell my family because they would worry, once I did, I was overwhelmed by their response. Eric was spectacular and supportive, and there for me whenever I needed him. Both of my parents are gone, but my sister Sally, her husband Rich, and their three children were calling me, and stopping by to see me, and generally just letting me know how much they loved me. Even my relatives by marriage, with whom I don't always see eye to eye, rallied around me. I only have a few close friends, but they, too, offered their love and support unconditionally. I mentioned before that I have always been somewhat of a loner, and it was, and is, humbling to realize the warm and beautiful understanding that I am loved and cared for. It changed my attitude about my connection with my family and my friends, and made me realize in a very positive way that yes, I'm an individual, but within a strong network of community. That realization made me feel healthy in a way I had never experienced.

STEP 1: Preparation for Surgery

You mean I get free liposuction? Let's do that!

(My comment to the plastic surgeon when choosing what kind of surgery to have.)

(See Rule #1)

My diagnosis had been in late February, and so it was early March when I met with the surgeon to talk about my options. There were two types of surgery I could have. My surgeon insisted that I talk to the plastic surgeon and discuss them before I made a final decision, just so I'd know everything about each procedure and each outcome. So I met with the plastic surgeon. He was a serious, sad-faced man, who had what I've dubbed "The Cancer Face" on. When he entered the room, he put his hand on my arm and said, "I'm so sorry you are going through this." Although it was very thoughtful, and I'm sure he was sincere, it was a little odd; he was a total stranger, and he seemed more upset than I was.

Option one was a total mastectomy and reconstruction. It was an extensive surgery. When the plastic surgeon described it to me, it sounded horrible. An overnight stay, plus a drainage tube for a few weeks. And later there would be more incisions and healing time as part of the reconstruction. The plastic surgeon seemed to like the idea of the total mastectomy, but when queried, it turned out that the reason was that he felt he could control the aesthetics of the outcome better. They (the surgeon and the accompanying nurse, who had had that exact procedure done) went on to explain that with a total mastectomy, an implant is put under the pectoral muscle and slowly inflated. When I asked about permanent restrictions on exercise, the nurse said, "Well, pushups would be out." After all the hard work I had done already with my workouts and how good they were making me feel, my response to that was, "Well, then let's not go with that." I don't think they understood how important it was to me to be able to continue my regular exercise. It was crucial to my physical and mental health. I also didn't like the idea of a foreign object being put in my body if it wasn't absolutely necessary. I would've done it if I had had to, of course, but I didn't have to.

Option two was a lumpectomy, removal of some lymph nodes, and follow-up radiation. It was an outpatient procedure: I could have the surgery on Friday and go back to work on Monday. With the lumpectomy, of course, my right breast would be smaller. The plastic surgery solution to that? Liposuction fat from another part of my body and fill it in. I couldn't help thinking how elegant an idea that was – using the body's own cells to minimize rejection. I also liked the natural approach of that method. The surgeon warned me that he wasn't sure he could make it look like it had before. I didn't care. When I said "You mean I get free liposuction? That's a bonus!" neither he nor the nurse was in the least amused at my levity.

HOW ARE *THEY* FEELING?
My god, I know it's cancer, but does everyone have to be so damned dreary and serious?

RULE #2
Humor can be found – and often should be – in the most unlikely places.

I wasn't thrilled about the mastectomy option; that was major, invasive surgery. I also wasn't thrilled about the idea of radiation – I've spent my whole life trying to avoid getting X-rays – but I liked the idea of keeping my body as whole and as much like it had been before as possible. While I didn't want to be disfigured, it seemed the less invasive surgery was the best option for me. In fact, when I wrote in my journal about total mastectomy, my response was "Eww." They scheduled the surgery for mid-April.

<u>RULE #3</u>
No matter what the doctors and nurses recommend, remember that they have their own biases as well. Sort the facts, weigh your options, and choose what is right for you.

<u>INSIGHT</u>
I've spent my whole life nervous about all the things that I've read can increase your risk of cancer. Things like x-rays, sodium laureth sulfate, bacon (nitrites), bleached coffee filters (dioxin)…the list goes on and on. I used to say "I don't use/eat such-and-such; it's been linked to cancer. Now I say jokingly, "Better not do that; I might get cancer!" And then I just laugh. While I don't advocate throwing caution to the wind, and heedlessly using or eating these things, I'm certainly enjoying my bacon more. It does change your perspective. I'm not *afraid* of those things anymore.

<u>RULE #4</u>
Cancer can be liberating.

Once I knew what I was facing, it was time to become proactive with my exercise and mind-body medicine. I was determined to get myself into the best physical shape and spiritual balance possible *before* having the surgery, so that I would not only recover more quickly, but also not stress about the whole thing. By coincidence, over the previous Christmas vacation I had made myself a chart of the activities I wanted to spend time on each week. This had included exercises and meditation, but I had only managed to achieve two to three workouts a week, and usually only two or three meditations. I knew that would not be enough. My experience with practicing music for most of my life has taught me that if you practice something every day, it becomes a way of life. That was what I needed: for these activities – exercise, meditation, guided imagery, etc. – to become a way of life. Also, once you've passed fifty (I was 57), exercise has to be more frequent than when you were in your twenties to get the same benefit. I felt that meditations and workouts would have to be at least five per week for either to have a major impact. So I revised my chart, and this is an example of what I used:

Meditation - 1/2 Hour						
Exercise - 1/2 Hr Walking/running						
Exercise - 1 Hour Yoga						
Guided Imagery/Affirmations						

I'd put X's in the boxes at the end of each day, and by the end of the week, it would look something like this:

Meditation - 1/2 Hour	X	X	X	X	X	X
Exercise - 1/2 Hr Walking/running		X		X		
Exercise - 1 Hour Yoga	X		X		X	X
Guided Imagery/Affirmations	X	X	X	X	X	

Finding a time to work out has always been a challenge. I am a self-employed musician. I teach a few classes at a local community college, teach private lessons in my home, and perform locally. This makes my schedule sometimes different every week, and it makes it hard to find exercise classes to go to. Many of them are in the early morning or the evening, both teaching times for me. I have had to do virtually all of my exercising on my own.

I looked at my schedule and figured out where I could fit in the workouts. No more of this "I don't have time," or "I hate to work out in the morning". I *had* to make time, even if I had to get up earlier – and I *hate* getting up early. But I did. Monday, Wednesday and Friday I would do an hour of yoga (I already had a great DVD), and Tuesday and Thursday were aerobic exercise days. Any sort of aerobics would do; sometimes I took a brisk walk, sometimes I jogged, sometimes I exercised to a YouTube video to mix it up a little. Saturday and Sunday were bonus days, when I could work out if I wanted to, or use them as make up days if I'd missed one. The more I exercised, the more I enjoyed it, and the more I missed it when I didn't do it.

After each workout I would take about ten to fifteen minutes to cool down, and it was then that I would do my guided imagery. I had never really done guided imagery before, but I understood how it worked. You mentally put yourself in a relaxed, safe place, and you envision positive things happening. During my cool-down I would imagine myself filled with pure white light; light that illuminated all the dark corners of my body where cancer cells might be hiding. Then I would envision my white bloods cells diligently rushing in, enveloping the cells and killing them. I specifically focused on my right breast, where the tumor was, and each time I did the imagery methodically imagined clearing it of cancer cells. In my mind I cleared the surrounding areas as well, in case it had spread. Then I would imagine my system clearing away the leftover debris and eliminating it, leaving my breast, and my body, free of cancer and full of light.

Later on I found some wonderful guided imagery CDs by **Belleruth Naparstek**[3] and found that her imagery was very similar to mine. She has CDs which feature guided imagery and **affirmations**[4] on a variety of topics. Most useful to me were the ones called *Stress* and *General Wellness*. She has one called *Fighting Cancer*, which I wasn't quite ready for yet, and another called *Chemotherapy*, which I *certainly* wasn't ready for. At this point, I steadfastly refused to think about chemotherapy. The question of chemotherapy would be answered by the results of my surgery. If the cancer had spread and I was looking at chemotherapy down the road, I would deal with that obstacle at the appropriate time. I was hoping it wouldn't come to that.

---

[3] People and book and CD titles in bold are in Appendix II – Resources.

[4] See the glossary for examples of some of the images and affirmations typical of these CDs I listened to.

After about three weeks of five to six workouts a week and all that positive thinking, I felt spectacular, the worry of my impending surgery notwithstanding. I felt strong and healthy, and my mood was positive and cheerful. I had even lost five pounds, which made me feel both physically and mentally healthier. I hadn't been overweight, but I had acquired a little extra padding over the years.

Of course, in addition to my workouts and guided imagery and affirmations, I made sure I meditated at least five times a week. The more regularly I did it, the easier it got. After about a week or two of almost daily meditation, I could tell my meditative state was deeper and more relaxed. I began to experience a deep inner peace that was stronger than I had ever felt before. Both my mood and my inner peace might seem ironic, considering what I was going through, but that was how I felt.

As I said, I had done some workshops and some studying about sound healing therapy. By coincidence I had started to read a book *before* my diagnosis called *The Healing Power of Sound* by the late **Dr. Mitchell Gaynor**. He was an oncologist who incorporated **Tibetan singing bowl** meditations into his mainstream practice. It wasn't a coincidence that I was reading about sound healing therapy, since I was trying to learn how to do it, but it did seem fortuitous (and timely) that I had inadvertently chosen a book by an oncologist. The book was fascinating, informative, and well-researched with documentation of studies of the healing properties of sound. It also contained some case studies of Dr. Gaynor's patients and how the singing bowls had improved their recoveries/outcomes. I purchased some, and often played them as part of my meditation. Two of my meditation CDs featured the bowls, and I listened to them the most often.

I also incorporated into my mediation sessions **toning** and chanting, drawing on some research that shows that these practices can aid in healing and spiritual balance.

<u>HOW ARE YOU FEELING?</u>
People who knew me and knew what I was facing would gently touch my arm and say "How are you feeling?" with sincere concern. I truly appreciated them asking, but the truth was, with all the positive and healthy things I was doing, my answer was "Better than I've felt in years!" My niece remarked on more than one occasion "You seem more like Aunt Julie these days."
And I *felt* more like myself. I used to say to myself *You should exercise more, you should meditate more, you should spend more time studying sound healing therapy.* But then I wouldn't do it, and I would feel like a failure, like I wasn't reaching my full potential. I now felt like I was being the person I had imagined I could be. It was great.

While I didn't want to join a cancer support group, I knew I needed a support team of my own, so I made a point of going to one mind-body healing session every other week or so, for any additional help they might provide. I would've gone every week, but it can get expensive, and of course, health insurance doesn't cover those kinds of treatments. So I went as often as I could afford. An added bonus was that being around people who understand the power of these therapies reinforced my belief that I was on the right track. One week I would go for a Reiki session, another **Reflexology**, and another sound healing therapy. Sound Healing is my personal favorite. Perhaps it's because I'm a musician, but of all the things I did, sound has had the most profound impact on me. Sound Healing practitioners use a combination of various instruments (see glossary), but they rely heavily on the singing bowls.

I went to **Salt Therapy** rooms too, and that was relaxing. However, later on during chemotherapy both the salt room own and my oncologist warned against it during treatment. Apparently there can be bad side affects.[5]

Every day I was doing something positive for my health and well-being. That in itself was empowering and helped to keep me in good spirits. If I'd done nothing, and put all my hope in doctors and procedures, I would've felt helpless, worried and scared. And, as I mentioned before, stress can weaken your immune system.

---

[5] From what I've read, there are currently no research studies to create guidelines for patients and clinicians about salt therapy treatments. But that's true for some of the other modalities I was using. For more discussion about this, see: http://journals.lww.com/academicmedicine/Abstract/2001/12000/Why_Alternative_Medicine_Cannot_Be_Evidence_based.11.aspx

STEP 2: Surgery

I am NOT letting surgery keep me from yoga!

So how to prepare for surgery? I knew that when the day came, I would be nervous and stressed, just like everyone is, no matter how calm and peaceful I had become in the previous six weeks. You're in an unfamiliar place with unfamiliar people, except for your surgeon, who you barely know, and you're putting your life in all of their hands. Nothing to be worried about! So I continued my meditation, guided imagery, sound healing therapy and exercise, but that was all I could do until the day of the surgery.

The surgery entailed removing the tumor and the surrounding tissue (the "margins"), and also what are called the "sentinel nodes." These are the lymph nodes that the breast drains to first. By checking them, they could determine if the cancer had spread.

<u>THOUGHTS</u>
Medical and scientific terminology has always fascinated me, and I loved the idea that someone had named these nodes "sentinels." It makes them seem more prestigious somehow. How charming – and how accurate.

The day of the surgery came, and sure enough, I was nervous and apprehensive. I suppose I should have been worried about what they would find, but no, I worried that something would go wrong, and I'd die on the operating table. Fear isn't rational; it's just fear.

From all my readings about sound healing therapy and **Music Therapy**, I knew that playing music before and during surgery can lead to better surgical outcomes and recovery[6]. So I armed myself with Eric's iPod and a set of headphones, and I

---

[6] See the "Resources" Appendix for **Dr. Alice Cash**, who has devised a set of headphones made specifically for use during surgery.

loaded my favorite singing bowls meditation CD onto it. If nothing else, it would distract me from worrying.

While I sat in the waiting room, and later in the prep room for the operating room, I listened to the CD. The result was amazing. As soon as I put the headphones on and starting hearing the sounds, all the bustle and fuss around me faded away as though it wasn't real. Everyone else was so energetic and intense, but I felt like I was floating and detached, and that the energy of that world couldn't touch me. I'm sure it helped that it was a CD that I had meditated to many times; I associated it with peacefulness. I was actually astounded at how well it worked. Even I hadn't quite believed it could make so profound a difference.

By the time they came to take me to the OR, I was dreamy, peaceful and relaxed. Then they gave me a mild sedative to prepare me, which helped too, and they told me later that when they wheeled me into the OR I was chatty and cheerful. I don't remember most of that, of course.

It was a long day, though. They sent me home in the late afternoon with pain meds, and I found that I didn't even need them. They had used glue to close the incisions – one on my breast and one between my breast and my right armpit – and as long as I moved carefully it didn't hurt.

<u>PROCEDURES INADVERTANTLY TURNED INTO ART</u>
They had injected my right breast with blue dye, so they could locate the sentinel nodes, and when I got home, looking in the mirror I saw the most beautiful blue swirly pattern on my breast. I wish I had taken a picture of it, it was so striking.
Of course, later I peed blue!

The surgery was on a Friday. Saturday I felt great, and still didn't need any pain medication. Many people thought I was crazy, but my plan was to resume yoga on Monday. I had gotten so used to exercise that I resented the surgery for taking me away from it.

When I look back through my journal, even I am

surprised at how optimistic I sounded. Here is what I wrote on Sunday, only two days after my surgery:

I live in a beautiful house in the country; I love my work, my music, my writing and my kitties. I am surrounded by people I love and who love me. Eric, Sally, Rich and the girls are so loving and supportive and I know they will continue to be. I feel like my life is wonderful.

INSIGHT
Way back when I had gotten my diagnosis, one of the nurses suggested I keep a journal, and although I had been keeping a journal for many years, I will always be grateful for her reminder about how therapeutic it can be. Recently studies have been done proving its positive impact.

RULE #6
Keep a journal. It helps to get your thoughts and feelings out, and you can say anything you want to *yourself*.

And so, because I couldn't live with myself if I didn't, I got up on Monday morning and did an hour of yoga. *Very* carefully. I had to do Downward Facing Dog one-handed, which was challenging, but not impossible. I had to modify some of the ways I stretched, but I did it, and I was thrilled and super pleased with myself. Like I said earlier, I've spent years, like many people, thinking I should exercise, meditate, take better care of myself, etc., but my implementation of that was spotty. I had been afraid the surgery would offer me an opportunity to slip back into old habits, but it didn't. I had a mission. The way I looked at it was that I was in training for my life.

Of course, brisk walking was easy to do; running was obviously out for a while. Starting with that Monday I returned to my regular routine of exercise, meditation, guided imagery, and other mind-body healing techniques. I added some additional imagery and thoughts about my body mending quickly and fully. Except for the handicap of not being able to stretch my right arm out completely, I felt perfectly normal, and it was only four weeks before I had full range of motion again.

When I returned to my surgeon for a follow-up appointment (after two weeks), she was impressed that I was doing so well, but alarmed that I had begun yoga so quickly again. I assured her I had been careful, but I was surprised that she didn't seem to make the connection between the two.

<u>THOUGHTS</u>
Throughout all of my treatments my healthcare professionals have been pleased at my quick recovery, but most of them have been dismissive, indifferent, or even alarmed at my activities. The Breast Center, where I got my initial diagnosis, seemed more supportive of this, or at least tolerant, but I wondered about the rest of the doctors and nurses. Were they not aware of the studies I'd been reading? Studies showing improved outcomes from careful exercise, meditation, guided imagery, and the use of music/sound have been around for decades. What is wrong with our healthcare system that this isn't part of a standard treatment plan?

Unfortunately, although the surgery and my recovery went spectacularly well, it turned out the cancer had spread to the sentinel nodes. This meant I would need a second surgery to remove more lymph nodes to see if it had spread any further. On a more positive note, the margins around the tumor had been clear, so no more surgery there. While I was not thrilled (to put it mildly) about the prospect of a second surgery, or the possibility that the cancer might have spread beyond the sentinel nodes, my response to the doctor and nurse was, "Yay, I get to keep my boob!" I don't think they quite knew what to do with me. To people who deal with breast cancer patients every day, the goal is – and should be – the best procedure to ensure total recovery. Lopping off breasts becomes routine for them, or at least that was the way it seemed to me from the way they behaved. For me, every instance where I didn't have to lose parts of my body or put foreign things in it was a cause for celebration. While this new development was scary, I was grateful for the positive side.

* * *

INTERLUDE – WHY AREN'T YOU SCARED?

By this time you are probably wondering how I managed to be so steadfastly upbeat. Didn't I *ever* freak out, cry, worry, stress? The answer is yes; I did all of those things. What would generally happen was that if I drank a couple of glasses of wine, my inhibitions would drop, my rational thoughts would fade, and I would have a little meltdown and a good cry. But honestly, over the course of a year of procedures and treatments, this only happened three or four times.

Here are the reasons I managed to remain cheerful and positive throughout all of my treatments. Some of these I have mentioned before, but I thought I'd list them. Think of it as your "To Do" list of how to keep a positive attitude and ward off stress and worry.

One: My husband Eric was always there for me. Once I had the initial diagnosis, he went to every doctor's appointment and procedure with me. We made sure to schedule them so this was possible. Just having him there was comforting and helped me to feel safe. In addition to Eric, the outpouring of love and support from my family and friends was overwhelming. *That* made me cry. As I mentioned, I like to spend a lot of time alone. Their support made me more aware of my place in a community, and that changed my view of my life and the people in it in a beautiful, positive way.

> **MESSAGE**: Have someone to hold your hand, no matter what. If you don't have an "Eric," take a friend or relative, or find a cancer support group and get a "buddy."

Two: Since Eric is a nurse practitioner, he was able to advise me when I didn't fully understand something, or couldn't remember all the details the doctor had mentioned.

His knowledge and research helped me to feel more certain that I was making the right choices.

MESSAGE: If you don't have someone close to you who knows something about healthcare, do your own research so you don't feel like you're just blindly following your doctors.

Three: Reminding myself that every treatment was *my* choice was empowering. I could have chosen not to have a mammogram in the first place, not to have the tumor removed, and not to have chemotherapy or radiation (which I'll get to later). The knowledge that *I* was choosing made me feel good about myself, and not like my life was out of control.

MESSAGE: Remember that you are in control of your choices. You have to live with the consequences, but *you* are in charge.

Four: Endorphins. I have no doubt that the endorphins my body was releasing from all the exercise helped to keep me happy. In fact, the few times I skipped a couple of days of exercise, I noticed that I began to worry, stress and feel more helpless. That certainly gave me the incentive to keep running and doing my yoga.

MESSAGE: Keep exercising. For your body *and* your mind!

Five: The meditations, affirmations and guided imagery were more helpful than you might imagine. They filled my mind with positive thoughts about healing and peacefulness. Plus, as I mentioned earlier, they (and the exercise) made me feel like every day I was doing something positive for my mind and body. For example, saying the words "More and more, I can stop worrying about things I cannot change, and focus on my own inner peacefulness" is a much better thing to say over and over to yourself than "Oh my god, what if they find more cancer?" Likewise, saying "I accept assistance from my loved ones – past, present and future – and I feel myself surrounded by their love and caring. I can feel it all over my body like a warm wave" beats "Shit, what am I gonna do?"

The worst time was probably late at night when I was trying to go to sleep. If I felt troubled, I would listen to some affirmations, or better yet, one of Belleruth's CDs called *Peaceful Sleep*. It is a guided imagery that helps distract you from negative thoughts.

MESSAGE: Focus on the positive aspects of your life, peacefulness, and the blessings that you have.

Six: In addition to nurturing my mind and spirit, supplementing my conventional treatments with Reiki and sound healing therapy was extremely helpful. After my sessions I would feel peaceful, balanced and healthy. I don't know exactly how they work – which is part of the reason the mainstream medical community doesn't embrace them – but I have experienced profound changes with these two therapies in particular. Even if it's "all in my mind," if it makes me healthier, that's a good thing. We've been taught "all in your mind" is a negative thing, but think about it for a minute: its common knowledge that you can make yourself sick. If that's true, then you can make yourself well, too. If it works one way, it works the other. We have the power to help heal ourselves.

However, I believe that Reiki and sound Healing *do* have a positive effect. We just don't know how to measure it very well yet.

MESSAGE: If something works to make you healthier, happier, etc., keep doing it and ignore the eye-rollers.

Seven: While I don't have a "bucket list", the one thing I had wanted to do for years was move back to the country. I grew up in the country, and when Eric and I moved in together, we moved to the city of Harrisburg, PA, because it was cheaper. What with career challenges and helping to take care of my handicapped mother, we ended up living in the city for thirty years. Then we bought an acre of land, built our own house, and moved in.

I was so happy. I felt like I was home again after years of being away. It was only six months after we moved in that I got my diagnosis. I would wake up in the morning with the birds chirping, look out the window and see the stretches of trees and farmland and think, "This is so awesome. I can't really complain. If I have to die, at least I can die here in this beautiful place."

> **MESSAGE**: Have something bigger that eclipses day to day worries. For me, being close to nature again was bigger than having cancer.

Eight: I wrote in my journal almost every night. What I said in Rule #6 was true; it helped me to get out thoughts and feelings that maybe I didn't want to talk about, or talk about too much to other people. It helped me to process those feelings. I would also put my completed charts in my journal at the end of the week, and I would write about what a good job I was doing with my exercise and alternative therapies. That would boost my spirits and remind me of the positive impact I was having.

> **MESSAGE**: Journaling can be amazingly therapeutic.

Nine: For years I had wanted to:
- get myself on a regular schedule of exercise
- meditate regularly and become more spiritual and peaceful
- get involved in some mind-body therapies and continue my study of sound healing therapy, with the thought of doing it for others some day

I had never been consistent about any of these things, and constantly berated myself for not reaching my full potential in these areas. And suddenly, here I was doing it. The diagnosis and treatments had galvanized me in a way that nothing else had. So even in the face of dire consequences, I felt like I was being the person I had always wanted to be. I was proud of myself. Part of my brain was saying "Yay, me!"

MESSAGE: We're all going to die. Be your full self while you are here.

Ten: I mentioned my mother previously. I watched her weather fifty-one years of MS, and throughout she was stubborn, strong, determined and optimistic. It never occurred to me that there was any other way to be. Her message, by example was, "Yes, I've got something that could kill me or seriously debilitate me, but it's just one of those things that can happen to you, like chronic back pain, or diabetes, heart failure, or arthritis. You accept it and move on and live. You can either see the glass as half empty or half full."

MESSAGE: If you have good role models, you have an advantage from the beginning. If you don't have any, seek them out!

Eleven: I kept reminding myself: *You could get hit by a bus tomorrow, or blown up in a terrorist attack, or die of a heart attack. At least you don't live in Syria, or any of these other places where people are suffering. I am not suffering like that.*

MESSAGE: Keeping perspective is extremely important. Always try to look at your situation from different angles.

* * *

STEP 3: Surgery #2

*Okay, getting back to yoga this time is going to be harder,
but I'm going to do it. It worked so well the first time…*

Because there was (as the doctors so charmingly put it)
"lymph node involvement," before my second surgery I was
sent for an MRI of my torso, plus a full body bone scan, to see
if there were any other tumors in my body. This made
everyone in my family extremely nervous because they were
afraid it had spread. It made me extremely nervous because
I've always had an irrational fear of procedures. Plus, I'm
claustrophobic.

I kept reminding myself of the tools I had gained over
the past weeks, and I put them to full use. When I got the bone
scan I couldn't listen to headphones because the machine was
going to come very close to my head. (Eeek! – that's where the
claustrophobia kicks in) So Eric read poetry to me. At
moments when he couldn't, I hummed quietly to myself, a
little meditational tune that I had devised.

I couldn't take Eric into the MRI with me, so I hummed
all the way through that scan as well. Sometimes I would just
tone on a single note. In both cases it calmed me and
distracted me from my fears.

<u>INSIGHT</u>
**I knew there was research that shows that mothers singing and
humming to their babies is therapeutic and helps with growth and
development, but I never fully appreciated how soothing it can be just
to hum to yourself.**

<u>RULE #7</u>
When you have no other resources, hum.

Of course I, too, was apprehensive about what they
might find, but as good as I felt, it was hard to imagine that
my body was riddled with tumors. It only took five days for

the results to come back. The nurse coordinator called me, and in that delightfully impassive clinical way they have, told me "You have no metastatic disease." (Meaning that it hadn't spread any further) I was relieved, to say the least. Everyone else in the family heaved a collective sigh of relief, and that evening Eric whipped out a bottle of champagne for a toast. I think he was more scared than he let on. (This was actually true of him the whole time. He tried to seem neutral through all the proceedings so I wouldn't worry more, but I knew it was hard for him.)

<u>BONUS</u>
While I didn't enjoy the procedures, afterwards I thought *How cool and reassuring to know that my body is clear of tumors. How often do you get this chance?* I don't mean because of the fear of spreading; I mean, how many times have you wondered if you have a tumor growing and you don't know about it? It was reassuring because of my lymph node involvement, but also just to know nothing was starting anywhere else. People without cancer can't just go for tumor scans unless they pay for it themselves. As you can imagine, it's pretty pricey. My insurance forms for that day added up to just under $10,000. Heck, I can get a facelift for less than that.

The second surgery was more extensive. It was called an "axillary node dissection." That is a procedure where they take out pretty much all of the lymph nodes under your arm. This allows them to check and see if the cancer has spread past the sentinel nodes.

The surgeon had warned me that while it was scheduled as outpatient surgery, it was four hours long, and patients sometimes had to stay overnight afterwards. Of course, I was convinced I would come through with no problems. I prepared in the same way I had done for the first surgery, and was sure to bring the iPod and listen to the singing bowls CD in the OR waiting room prior to my surgery.

The surgery took only three hours, and after three hours in recovery I was ready to go home. When the resident came in to check on me he stopped dead in his tracks, stared incredulously and said "You're dressed!"

"Yeah, I'm going home," I replied. "I feel fine." They were all totally impressed.

The second surgery was also on a Friday, and I was planning again to resume my yoga the following Monday. This recovery was a little more difficult. I finally broke down on Saturday and Sunday and took some of the pain medication they had given me, but Monday morning I was determinedly back on my yoga mat with no medication. It would've been a reasonable time to take a week off, but I persisted, even if I had to leave some of the yoga moves out. It was more complicated, too: I had a drainage tube for fluid under my right arm, which emptied into an attached bag. It was bulky and bumped against my side under my arm. But I managed to do my yoga! *Very* carefully. When I did inverted poses I held my arm against my body to stabilize the bag, and used only one hand to hold myself up. The drainage tube was painful, but as long as I moved slowly and carefully I was able to do a modified routine. Running was, once again, out for a while, but brisk walking was not much of a problem.

I worked out five days a week with modifications for three weeks until the drainage bag and the tube were removed, all the while maintaining my schedule of meditation, guided imagery, affirmations, Reiki and sound healing therapy. By three weeks I had regained some of my range of motion, but not as much, as the damage was more extensive. The surgeon had written me a prescription for Physical Therapy, and soon after the tube was removed, I went. The therapist helped my range of motion with some additional exercises, although she was quite impressed with how far I had already come. Some of my yoga stretches were actually better than her recommendations, so she told me to keep doing those. The truly amazing thing she did was to massage the scar and break up the scar tissue. Not only did this give me better flexibility, but it significantly improved the appearance of the scar. No puckering or wrinkling. You can barely see it, although it is six inches long.

I will forever be grateful to the surgeon for writing that script. Apparently, not all doctors do. I've talked to other breast cancer patients with similar surgeries whose doctors didn't. While my yoga stretches would have eventually given me close to full range of motion, breaking up the scar tissue made my arm and shoulder nearly as flexible as it had been before the surgery. And now, a year and a half later, my right and left sides are equally flexible. There's a little pulling on the scar site, but it doesn't interfere with my movement.

CURIOSITY
No one told me this would happen, but I noticed one day when I was working out that only my left armpit was sweating. The right was dry. Why? It turns out that when you cut all those nerves it impairs your ability to sweat. It was, and still is, a little weird, although over time it's improving.

A few weeks after the surgery I had a follow-up appointment, and the news was – I thought – pretty good. Only two of the fifteen lymph nodes they had removed had had cancer in them, and only a small bit. I would've been surprised if they had all been clear, and to me, a "small bit" was a sign that it hadn't spread further. However, this meant that they were recommending chemotherapy, which is what I had feared all along. Although it turns out that with the sentinel node involvement, they would've recommended it

anyway. So the surgeon made me an appointment with one of
the oncologists to discuss her recommendations.

STEP 4: Chemotherapy: First Half

I've been teaching Music Appreciation for twenty years. I've taught it with migraines; I've taught it with hangovers. I can teach it on chemotherapy.

(My thoughts when deciding not to take the fall semester off from teaching college during chemo. For some reason, people thought this was funny when I said it.)

The chemotherapy was a tough decision to make. From the very first moment of my diagnosis, every time the subject came up I would say "I might not do it." At first I think I was just dismissing it because it wasn't a decision I had to make yet. I had to deal with the surgeries and results first before I was ready to think about it. When it began to look like they were going to recommend it, I think it was a way for me to remind myself that it was still my choice.

It was my surgeon who had recommended chemotherapy to me, and had referred me to an oncologist at the same hospital. Because it was such a scary decision to make, for this phase I wanted to get a second opinion. Not only did I want to make sure that most oncologists would have the same recommendations, but I really wanted to find an oncologist that I felt comfortable with and trusted. Weirdly enough, I ended up getting the "second" opinion first. I didn't care for that oncologist at all. She seemed cold, detached, and hard to relate to.

I then went to the oncologist the surgeon had referred me to. She recommended the same treatment plan as the first had, which reassured me that the recommendations I was getting were generally agreed upon. I felt pretty comfortable with her. It was important to me to be with someone I could be open with about the other things I was doing as a complement to standard treatment. While she didn't seem to think they would do any good, at least she didn't roll her eyes.

I think she thought if it would make me feel better, it couldn't do any harm. That was good enough for me.

One of the first things I asked her was if the hospital was doing anything along the lines of alternative or complementary therapies. Not surprisingly, the answer was no. I asked if there was at least a nutritionist I could consult in-house, and when she said "No," at least she had the grace to look embarrassed. (They did give me a pamphlet on nutrition, but it didn't provide me with the level of depth I had hoped.)

<u>THOUGHTS</u>
While the hospital I went to is famous and well-respected, they've been very slow to incorporate holistic health practices. I know there are hospitals and facilities – Cancer Centers of America, to name a prominent one – that have begun using Complementary and Alternative Medicine (CAM), but it's still rare. I looked into Cancer Centers of America, but it wasn't in my insurance network. I couldn't afford to pay for of all this on my own. (More on costs later)

My oncologist recommended a course of eight chemotherapy treatments. One every two weeks for a total of sixteen weeks.

I really, really, really didn't want to do it. Who would? There were a lot of icky side effects – weakened immune system, nausea, fatigue, numbness, mouth sores – the list went on and on, and those were just side effects while you were in treatment. There were risks of problems after I finished treatment – permanent heart problems, neuropathy…well, you get the idea. In fact, here is what I wrote in my journal:

Chemo is evil. It's not so much the hair thing; it's the insult to my body. Are we still this barbaric? That we have to kill good cells in order to kill bad cells?

Of course, some of it *was* the hair thing. But I knew vanity could not be a factor in my decision. I was told that the statistics of people with similar staging and surgeries showed that chemotherapy would significantly reduce my chance of recurrence. That was a powerful argument. I also realized that if I didn't do it, I would spend the rest of my life worrying whether I should have, and whether the cancer was going to come back. So I said yes.

The first thing they did was send me to have a mediport installed. This is a clever little device that's surgically placed under your skin (for me above my left breast) and connects to a vein so they can give you your infusions. That way you don't have to have an IV in your arm for a couple of hours during treatments. It was at once creepy and fascinating. It was kind of exotic to have this sophisticated medical thing in me. Sounds weird, but it's true. Then all I had to do was await my first treatment.

<u>THOUGHTS</u>

Once I had decided to do the chemo, I had to make a choice about whether or not to take the fall semester off from teaching class. I knew other people who had taken a hiatus from work for chemo, and wondered if it would be wise to do so. The quote at the beginning of this section notwithstanding, the more I thought about it the more I realized that if I took the time off, *I would just sit around with lots of time to feel scared and sick*. That would not do. Besides, I love my job and my life. The best thing for me to do was to keep living it as much like normal as possible.

So how was I going to prepare for something like *this*? I knew I would be terrified when I went to the infusion center, particularly the first time. So I started collecting talismans. I asked everyone in my immediate family to give me something of theirs that I could take with me, so that they would "be there" with me. From my three nieces I received a bracelet, a cherished stuffed dog from childhood, and a piece of rose quartz (supposedly a crystal of unconditional love). Sally and I had nearly matching necklaces that she previously had had made for us, and we both wore them constantly. Even some of my piano students donated items. These tokens of love and support comforted me more than you can possibly imagine. I kept them in a small box and took them with me every time I went for a treatment, sometimes putting them out on a table where I could see them.

I had been keeping up with my five-day-a-week exercise routine (of course!), and I worried about how well I would be able to keep that up. So the morning of my first treatment I got up early and did my yoga, so I wouldn't miss that day. I knew I couldn't afterwards. Looking back, even I can't believe I had the drive to do that. I've never been good at getting up early to exercise. But it was empowering, and so I did it.

I won't pretend that I wasn't terrified when I went to the hospital for my first infusion. I knew they would be filling my body with horrible, toxic chemicals that would make me feel awful. I kept telling myself that it would kill the cancer cells, and that was a *good* thing, and that it was temporary.

Of course, Eric came with me, and I took my recordings of the singing bowls. The first thing they did was give me steroids and anti-nauseants, so the chemo wouldn't make me throw up (a pleasant thought). When it came time for the infusion of the chemo drugs, I turned on the iPod, selected the singing bowls CD tracks, put the headphones on, and drifted into my meditational world. I steadfastly refused to look at the IVs, or anything else that would remind me of where I was and what was happening. It wasn't fun, but the sound of the bowls was soothing and made me think good, relaxing thoughts about harmony and balance – things larger than that single moment.

<ins>INSIGHT</ins>

It really helped to think of my life as a continuum, instead of an individual moment. I actually learned this trick from being a musician. I learned that if I focused on each individual performance – right now – I was more likely to suffer from stage fright. (Which has been an issue for me) But if I thought about each single performance as one in a long line of gigs that I would play over my lifetime, that are part of my growth as a musician, each individual event wasn't as scary.

<u>RULE #8</u>
Sometimes it's important to live in the moment. Sometimes it serves you better to focus on the larger picture.

I didn't feel that bad afterwards. It took a couple of days for it to really hit me, which, I had been told, was typical. The experience was mostly just scary. So I went home and waited to see what would happen. Eric actually took me out to dinner that evening to make life seem more normal.

The infusion was on a Friday, and by Sunday I was feeling pretty awful. However, I managed to do my yoga routine. I realized very quickly that running would not be an option – much too tiring – but I could do brisk walking. That first week I managed three yoga workouts and two brisk walks. It felt very good and positive, and I thought *I can do this. I'll be all right.*

<u>BONUS</u>
Once I started the treatments, Sally insisted on bringing me (and Eric) homemade soup every Friday, even though I only had a treatment every other Friday. This small gesture was a constant reminder of her support and caring: a way for her to do something positive toward my healing and recovery. You wouldn't imagine that a mason jar of soup can emanate love, but it did. Every spoonful was a reminder that she was with me, thinking about me. She told me later, too, that it was a way that *she* could feel like she was helping me heal. And she was.

<u>RULE #9</u>
Don't turn gifts away. It's easy to say "Oh, you don't have to bother," or "I'll be okay." Accept the gifts that people offer you. It means something to you *and* them.

In that first week I started to get sores in my mouth, which worried me a little. I was told that once you get them it's hard to get rid of them. I also quickly learned that there were foods that would irritate my mouth, even if they had never done so before. Salsa and olives in particular, balsamic vinegar, and anything very spicy were off the list. Wine was a little irritating as well, which was sad. I do like a glass of good

Chardonnay. My oncologist had recommended Orajel, an over the counter remedy for mouth sores, but one of my chemo nurses had told me that gargling with salt water and baking soda would help, or sucking on ice. I avoided the irritating foods, gargled with the salt water and baking soda, and the sores went away. They never bothered me after that.

Sadly, there were also foods that just plain tasted awful. Veggie burgers, one of my staples, tasted like cardboard. The worst tragedy of all was chocolate. Often my afternoon snack had been a square or two of dark chocolate. Yes, I *can* eat just one or two. As an adult I've never had much of a sweet tooth, but I love dark chocolate. It tasted *terrible*. And of all times to want comfort food and not be able to stand it. After all, chocolate keeps the dementors[7] away, and I was surrounded.

Actually, I did develop a bit of sweet tooth during that time, and at least was able to eat milk chocolate and enjoy it. It was better than nothing.

The second week I also managed two brisk walks and three days of yoga workouts. Of course I was continuing my meditation, my work with the singing bowls, my guided imagery and my affirmations, and was quite pleased at how it all helped to keep my spirits up. No doubt the endorphins from the exercise helped.

Of course, I wondered when my hair would start falling out. Every day I would get up, go into the bathroom and tug at my hair. It took just under two weeks. The day before my second treatment I took a brush to my hair in the morning and big clumps fell out. It was quite a spectacular sight. That was a Thursday. It wasn't too noticeable for a day or two, and I didn't have to go to any public places where I would be seen, but by Sunday I thought *No sense in trying to hide this or pretend it isn't happening. Let's get it over with.*

---

[7] Harry Potter fans (of which I am an avid one) will recognize dementors as evil creatures who suck all the happiness from the room you are in, or in extreme cases, suck out your soul. They guard the wizarding prison Azkaban. Chocolate keeps them at bay, or at least helps you to recover from their effects.

So Sally, who is very good at cutting hair, came over and she trimmed it a little at a time to different lengths to see what different hairstyles would look like on me, just for fun. Once we got it really short, Eric shaved the rest off with his shaving razor. We took pictures of the whole process, I suppose because it was so momentous.

I was 58, and had had long straight hair since I had been in eleventh grade. I grew up in the 1960s and 70s, and long hair meant you were cool. Not only that, but as a musician; my long hair was part of my image as a folk-rock acoustic singer/songwriter. My sense of identity and how I imagined people perceived me was so intertwined with my hair, as I'm sure it is for most people, that it was going to be very frightening to lose that part of myself. I looked on the Internet for head shaving rituals, thinking I might find something to help me through the transition. Unfortunately, everything I found was really weighty, like offering up your hair to Kali, making it sound very solemn and sacred. That was a little over the top for me. I finally just thought *After all, it's only hair. It'll grow back. This is the least of my worries.*

So I wrote a silly poem to read to Eric and Sally, which I read before he shaved my head. Here it is:

The Head-Shaving Poem

So now I'm going to shave my head
But I'm not really fussed
At least I will not worry
About it being mussed

Morning preparation will be
simple and sublime
Just pull my hair on, grab my coat
no extra wasted time

Ann was flabbergasted
when I said I'd lose my hair
She thinks I'm such a badass
that the chemo wouldn't dare

But this affects most everyone
the lowbrows and the highbrows
Heck, I'll just be happy if
I get to keep my eyebrows

And it's an opportunity
to see how I'm perceived
by other people and myself
I really can't be peeved

My ego and self-image
for so many years, you know
have been tied to this appearance
it's time to let it go

I both relish it and loathe it
on that you can depend
But I know that I'll be wiser for it
when I reach the end

I have the opportunity
to try out some new things
It would not have been my first choice
but let's see what it brings

Besides my chiropractor said
"You'll totally rock the bald thing"[8]

Sally laughed and laughed, which was fun. I think it

8 Feel free to copy or share this with anyone, if you think it will lighten their day.

was harder for them than it was for me, and the poem helped. And as weird as it was to look in the mirror and see myself bald, I really meant what I said in the poem. I'd been locked into the same self-image for so long – maybe even trapped by it – that this was an opportunity to shake things up and look at myself in a different way. That realization really helped me to put a positive spin on what was inevitable. And actually, it was kind of refreshing to have no choice but to change. I know many women change their hair color and style all the time, but I had always been afraid to. Plus, it did end up being pretty hassle-free: no fussing with my hair in the morning, no trying to find the best shampoo to make my slightly thinning hair look thicker. It certainly had its upside. Yoga was easier, too.

The American Cancer Society offers free wigs to chemo patients, and I had gotten one. I thought I would use it. The idea of wearing a turban, or one of those perky hats with no hair peeking out from underneath, seemed like I was screaming to the world "I'm on chemotherapy," and I vowed I wouldn't do it. But once I was bald, I hated the wig. The wig felt like I was pretending to be normal, and the turban felt more like I was owning it. So I bought some really cool scarves and learned to tie them into turbans (with some help from YouTube). I took special care with my makeup, and kept wearing earrings only in my left ear (a signature look of mine for many years), only now it was really obvious, since my hair didn't cover it up.

I didn't think much about it; I just wanted to still look pretty in the mirror, but I was unprepared for some of the responses I got:

– A few times, total strangers would say to me something like, "Oh, I love your look!"

– One of my students from college said, "Oh, that look suits you; it's artsy and exotic."

– I ran into a former student (a young wanna-be rocker), who said, "Wow, I wouldn't have the balls for that." He thought I had shaved my head as a statement. A reminder to me that some people do shave their heads because they *want* to.

- And then there were people I met who had never seen me before the cancer, who when they saw me after my hair started growing back in, said "I didn't realize you were on chemo. I just thought that was your style."

- The custodial staff at my college told me later they would talk together and wonder what kind of cool turban Julie was going to be wearing that day. "Did you see the one she has on today?" Miss Betty would ask Miss Linda. "It's so pretty." They told me they thought I looked so beautiful. That was a real shock to me. For the first time in my life, I had become glamorous.

<table>
<tr><td align="center"><u>RULE #10</u>
Never assume you know what people are going to think of you.
You're seldom right.</td></tr>
</table>

My favorite turban was a scarf my niece Carolyn loaned me. She is a Reiki Master and had recently gone to a guided meditation with some Buddhist monks. She had purchased the scarf there, and it had been blessed by one of the monks. When I wore it, I always thought about how she loved me, and the intent of the blessing. It felt very special, and I felt special wearing it, like it was a talisman. It also reminded me that some people – in this case monks – shave their heads for spiritual reasons.

<table>
<tr><td align="center"><u>CURIOSITY</u>
Everyone knows that your hair falls out when you do chemotherapy. Lesser known, or thought about, is the fact that all your hair stops growing. People said to me, "You mean your eyelashes fell out?" I didn't want to breach decorum and mention, well, unmentionable areas, so I responded, "Yeah, nose hair, too. Who knew?" I also never realized how much I relied on my eyelashes to guide my hand when putting on eyeliner. I had to completely retrain myself, after the last lashes were almost all gone and I started accidentally drawing wiggly lines on my cheeks. Luckily I am blessed with thick bushy eyebrows, which never completely went away.</td></tr>
</table>

By the time I was facing my third chemo infusion, four weeks in, my spirits were beginning to flag a bit. I could tell my body was getting weaker, and exercising was becoming more taxing. Also, now that I had done it twice, I knew what to expect: when I would start feeling crappy, and how it would affect my energy. On top of that, the following Monday I was scheduled to start fall classes at the college where I teach. I was a little apprehensive about how well I would weather that. Although I was looking forward to teaching, I wasn't looking forward to facing my colleagues and three full classes (approx. 100 students) with my new "turban" look. I wondered what they'd think, and I didn't want to have to talk about it and explain it to everyone.

One of my adult piano students, a woman in her forties, asked how I was feeling when she came to her lesson that week. She was a nurse's aide, and was interested in my progress, so I felt comfortable sharing details with her. When I lamented that I had only had the energy to exercise three times that week, she said, "Well, that's three more times than I did!" That helped my attitude considerably. I was exercising more than someone who *wasn't* on chemotherapy. It was a reminder that I was proactively influencing my health with my attitude and all my complementary modalities. They were the only weapons I had, but as I was learning, they were powerful ones.

IT'S WORKING!

Yes, I felt weak and things tasted bad, but apparently I was weathering the chemo very well. When I had gone in for my second treatment, my oncologist was very impressed with how well I was doing. I had to meet with her each time; they always send you for blood work the day of your treatment to check things like your white and red blood cell count, your liver enzymes, and your kidney function before they'll give you another treatment. If your numbers are bad, sometimes they postpone the treatment. Mine, while not stellar, were within the normal range. Even Eric, who's an NP, said "Are you sure they're giving you enough?" He couldn't believe how well I was doing. He's seen many patients on chemo, and most of them had not done as well.

The whole process of getting chemotherapy is more complex than I had realized. It's not just the chemo drugs; they give you a whole rash of pills and infusions. They gave me steroids and anti-nauseants the day of my infusion, and then I was to take them for two more days afterwards. I also had to go in the day after chemo and get a Neulasta shot. This is a drug that helps boost your white blood cell count. So I'd get my treatment on Friday, and on Saturday and Sunday, I'd feel pretty good, partly because the effects of the chemo drugs hadn't kicked in yet, but also because I was high on steroids. By Monday and Tuesday I'd start to feel awful, but I had to wonder how much of that was due to coming down off the steroids. On the other hand, I never experienced any nausea at all, for which I was quite grateful.

<u>THOUGHTS</u>

I said I'd return to money later. I mentioned that one reason I didn't go to the Cancer Treatment Centers of America was that it was out of my healthcare network, and I couldn't afford to pay for it myself. The wisdom of that decision became starkly clear when I started getting my "This is not a bill" statements from my insurance company. The scans, the surgery, the chemo were stunning in how expensive they were. The most spectacular fee, without a doubt, was the Neulasta shots. $14,000 each. I had eight of them; one for each treatment. That alone comes to $112,000. Yikes! Luckily I have excellent health insurance, but I've read horror stories about people who stop their treatments because they can't pay for them, and if they die, don't want to leave their families saddled with their debt. Another reminder that things could've been far worse.

I've mentioned that I didn't have too many meltdowns during my entire cancer treatment, but I did have a few. One of them came the week after my third infusion. By the Wednesday after my treatment I felt terrible. So bad, in fact, that I felt an overwhelming desire to crawl out of my own body, out of that space of toxicity. I wanted to claw at my skin and dig myself up out of the pit of poisonous chemicals I was awash in. It was one of the most uncomfortable feelings I've ever had, even though I had no real pain. I thought, *This is wrong, wrong, wrong. I can't do it anymore.*

After that experience, when I met with my oncologist for the fourth treatment, I expressed my feeling that maybe I would quit. My numbers were still okay from my blood tests, but my positivity was fading. I could *feel* how toxic I was. My oncologist was not pleased at the prospect. She looked me directly in the eye and said "If your cancer comes back, you will die."

I knew that she was speaking from probabilities based on statistics, and that it might not be true for me, but it certainly had the dramatic effect she intended. Ultimately, I chose to continue for two reasons: One, her statement reminded me that I had agreed to do this so I wouldn't spend the rest of my life worrying if the cancer was going to come back. If I quit, I would worry a lot more. Two, the treatment plan they had put me on were for four infusions of Adriamycin and Cytoxan together (just sounds icky, doesn't it?), and then four infusions of Taxol – eight treatments in all. She assured me that I wouldn't feel as tired on the Taxol. (Although as I discovered, it had its own debilitating side effects.) I thought, okay, I can do the first drugs one more time. Then we'll see how I stand the Taxol.

So I did the fourth infusion. The week after, I actually managed to do yoga twice, which pleased me greatly. On the other hand, someone had given me a small lilac seedling, and I went outside and planted it. Even that small act of digging a little hole so overtaxed me that I got quite dizzy, and when I was done I had to go inside and rest for a while. (The lilac, however, did fine and is still thriving.)

HOW DID I DO IT?

So how did I manage to maintain my yoga schedule in the face of that fatigue? By resting. I have a DVD routine that I've been doing for years. If I got tired anytime during it, I simply rested until I could keep going. Sometimes it took me an hour and fifteen minutes to do a fifty-five minute routine, but I didn't care. I knew it was good for me.

BONUS

My mother-in-law had been plagued for many years by a number of ailments. She'd been back and forth to doctors and was often on numerous medications. By the time she'd reached her early 70s, she was having trouble getting around, complaining of chronic pain, and seemed defeated. She couldn't prepare meals like she used to, and often went to bed early even if family was visiting. She spoke sometimes about how she might die soon, and how maybe that wouldn't be such a bad thing after all.

This went on for a few years, with some ups and downs, but around the time I was doing chemotherapy, three things happened that caused her to have a complete turn-around. One, Eric reviewed her medications and suggested some changes to get her off some of them. (In PA, nurse practitioners can prescribe medicine.) Two, he took her case and gave her a homeopathic remedy. (Remember he's also a classical homeopath.) Three, it turns out I completely inspired her. She emailed me one day about half way through my chemo and wrote, "I wanted to tell you what an inspiration you've been to me. I sit around complaining about all my aches and pains, and here you are going through chemo with your head held high. You refuse to let it stop you. Your example has inspired me to not let my health problems stop me from enjoying my life."

In the following months, in a way that seemed nearly miraculous, all of her symptoms got better. She became more mobile, more alert, and more engaged in her life with my father-in-law and the rest of their extensive family. She started cooking meals from scratch again, and now, a few years later, at 81, she's still going strong, and doing better than she has in years.

It may be that *all* of those things helped her, but it certainly helped to reinforce my belief in the power of positive thinking and the value of what I was doing. I thought *If my journey has helped to improve someone else's life dramatically, I am humbled and grateful that something good can come out of this. I know it has for me, but apparently for others, too.*

STEP 5: Chemotherapy: Second Half

Man, I am super high!

(My response to fifty milligrams of IV Benadryl.)

The Taxol was a new adventure entirely. A lot of people have allergic reactions to it – oh, goody, another thing to worry about – so the night before my infusion I was instructed to take twenty milligrams of Dexamethasone, a steroid, to help counteract any allergic reaction. Eric said twenty milligrams was a lot. They also gave me another twenty milligrams of Dexamethasone and fifty milligrams of Benadryl right before the infusion. That's a lot of Benadryl when you get it all at once, and I was really dizzy until the steroids kicked in and balanced it out a little. It was almost fun, once I got used to it. I figured they knew what they were doing and it wouldn't kill me, and after all, it wasn't like I was going to drive anywhere. I've never been much of a recreational drug taker, although I'm fond of Chardonnay, but I can appreciate a good buzz if I have no choice. I was also so high that I hardly cared about the chemotherapy drugs – an unintended positive side effect. With all that Benadryl on board, even with the steroids, I was feeling pretty loopy. The nurse thought it was really funny when I made the comment about being high.

That was on a Friday. By Sunday my hands were all red and puffy and I had a fever. Eric said it was erythrodysesthesia, or "hand-foot syndrome." This is a chemotherapy-induced condition that can include reddening, swelling, numbness and eventually peeling skin on the hands and/or feet, and sometimes the knees and elbows. It was really strange and uncomfortable. I was really tired, too. Monday came and I was still really tired. I managed to get through class, but after I got home I cancelled all my private music lessons, went to bed at 8:00 PM, and slept for twelve hours.

By Wednesday my hands were back to normal size. They did peel, but blessedly, they never swelled again throughout the next three treatments. I was very glad, because that condition can become very bad, and some patients have to halt their chemo in order to recover. Sometimes they have to switch drugs if it doesn't go away.

Once the allergic reaction was over, I felt pretty good. I had more energy than I had had on the first chemo drugs, and managed to work out four times that week, which really pleased me.

Another side effect that developed was my legs would twitch while I was sleeping, which would wake me up. Kind of like "restless leg syndrome," except, of course, it wasn't that. Taxol is toxic to the nerves, and this is a common side effect. Eric gave me a homeopathic remedy and it helped. It didn't completely relieve the symptom, but it abated the twitching enough that I could fall asleep. The twitching plagued me until well after the last treatment was over, but eventually passed.

Another unpleasant side effect of Taxol was numbness in my fingers and toes. They had told me this would happen. When I went in for my next treatment I mentioned it to my doctor and she said, "Can you write? Can you eat?" I thought *Holy shit, does it get that bad for some people?* Apparently so. I also mentioned that my feet were weak and numb, and she said "Can you walk?" I said yes, that it was only at night when I got up and had trouble going up the stairs. I was appalled at the thought of what other people must sometimes go through, and thought *All this stuff I'm doing must really be helping.*

An additional side effect to the Taxol was watering eyes. This became really annoying and messed up my eye liner, compelling me to check it regularly and reapply it frequently. I suppose I could've just stopped wearing it, but I was paying careful attention to how I dressed and did my makeup so that I would feel beautiful. It helped to keep my spirits up.

<u>RULE #12</u>
Never underestimate the positive effect of feeling you look your best.

Although the side effects were uncomfortable and scary sometimes, it could've been a lot worse. I purposely didn't read them because I knew it would freak me out. If there was anything good about the Taxol, it was that my taste buds improved, and food tasted a lot better.

By now you must be wondering how my work life was going through all of this. Pretty well, actually. I was teaching three classes that semester, and they were back-to-back. Every Monday, Wednesday and Friday I was in class from 10:00 AM to 1:00 PM. It was not taxing, but if I dropped something on the floor and leaned down to pick it up, I would get weak and dizzy when I stood up. A reminder that no matter how well I was doing, I still had a system full of poison.

Teaching piano and guitar lessons was easier: all I had to do was sit and listen, correct and praise. In fact, those were my best moments. I love teaching people how to play music, and I become so involved in it that the rest of the world goes away. So during lessons I was so absorbed by the moment that I would feel perfectly normal and forget I was on chemo.

I was very proud of the fact that I did not call in sick once throughout my entire chemotherapy regimen. I did cancel some of my private music lessons at home, but often I could just reschedule them to a different day. My students were understanding and flexible, and I appreciated it immensely.

However, I don't want to sugar-coat this. I did my work, and that was all. I went to bed around 9:30 every night and slept for many hours. I didn't practice the piano, guitar or singing, which was something I had always done regularly. I had thought I would catch up on my reading, but I didn't have the mental energy for that. I did crossword puzzles and read teen mysteries from my childhood. I had the energy for two things: 1) I kept at my regimen of all of the things I was doing to improve/maintain my health, and 2) I did the work I was obligated to.

Although I knew that meditation, sound healing therapy, Reiki, guided imagery, and other holistic and energy therapies can have wonderful positive effects on health, I must confess that throughout my surgeries and the early chemo, I suspected that the yoga and running (and then walking after chemo started) were doing more good than the other things. I knew from the past how good regular exercise made me feel, but hadn't had any experience with regular *daily* habits of the mind-body techniques. However, in the last weeks of chemo exercise became more and more difficult. I kept doing yoga and brisk walking, but they were wimpy workouts in comparison to what I had done before I began treatments. Still, I did what I could, because I knew every little bit helped.

It was then that I came to truly appreciate the positive benefits of the mind-body work I was doing. I continued to go for sound healing therapy and Reiki whenever I could afford it, and did guided imagery, affirmations and meditation on my own or with CDs on almost a daily basis. If I skipped a day, I could tell the difference. I would start to become depressed, despondent and worried. Most nights when I got into bed I would listen to dreamy meditation music or the *Peaceful Sleep* guided imagery CD. That helped me to drift off with pleasant thoughts in my head.

While I certainly didn't enjoy those last few weeks, it absolutely confirmed my belief in the therapeutic benefits the mind-body work provided me. In fact, I don't know how I would have endured without them.

<u>HAIR REVISITED</u>

So how did I feel after a couple of months wearing turbans? I had mixed feelings. Sometimes I'd look in the mirror at my bald head and get depressed. But I was aware that it wasn't just because I was bald; it was because of what the baldness represented. I actually liked my exotic look.

I still really appreciated the opportunity to be forced out of my perceptions of my identity. It was cleansing. I wanted my hair back, but I didn't want my old attitudes about my appearance back.

At the same time, I was also aware that when I *didn't* look in the mirror, I didn't care as much. Throughout the entire ordeal, I really became conscious of how I still felt like *me* on the inside. I thought looking different would change the way people thought about me, and I was afraid it would change the way I thought about myself. Of course, I did change, but in a good way. The things I was doing toward my own healing were very empowering for me. I felt like I was, and am now, a much better person.

I feel more flexible and daring with my looks. I feel like me on the inside, and I feel like I have more options for the outside.

The day of my last chemotherapy infusion was Halloween, just by a wild coincidence. Many of the nurses and staff at the hospital had dressed up for the occasion, which was fun. It certainly helped to lighten the mood in the infusion center.

There is a Starbucks in the medical center very close to the chemotherapy department, and before my infusion started I went over to get a cup of tea. As most of the people in line were staff, nurses, technicians, and doctors, some of them were dressed up, too. Of course I was wearing a turban, and in my left ear, as usual, I had long, dangly earrings. When my turn came in line, the clerk looked at me and said, "Oh, you're a gypsy!"

My immediate thought was, "No, you idiot, I'm a cancer patient. I'm only fifty yards from the infusion center." I didn't want to be rude, however, so I just mumbled "Sort of." Now, I look back on that moment fondly. I must've still looked healthy enough that she thought I was dressed up for Halloween.

<u>CHEMOTHERAPY CONCLUSION – SILVER LININGS</u>

- "Hair care" didn't exist. I didn't have to shave my legs or armpits, and I didn't have to fuss with my hair or buy shampoo. That sounds trivial, but after forty-plus years of doing those things, it was kind of liberating.

- Yoga was easier with a bald head. I even gave some thought (not much) to staying bald afterwards for the yoga benefits.

- I had the best excuse *ever* for not participating in things I felt obligated to do, but didn't really want to. Everyone understood when I didn't show up.

- Strangely enough, I felt safer while doing chemo. I felt like there was little chance that my cancer would recur during that time, so I didn't have to worry about that.

And the best…
- I learned that I didn't have to be perfect all the time, that I could be weak, and not always do my part, and my family and friends would still accept me and love me, and understand. What a wonderful feeling.

STEP 7: Chemotherapy recovery and into radiation – out of the fire into the frying pan.

The first thing on my mind after chemotherapy was "How long will it take me to feel normal again?" Of course, the answer is "never." You can't go through an experience like that without being changed irrevocably. Even if my body went back to "normal," which I didn't think it would completely, my mind was already different. That wasn't a bad thing. I've said all along that I liked the new ways I was thinking and acting. But of course I wondered how soon my body would restore itself. How long would it take my strength to come back? Once I had passed the two week mark (I'd been getting treatments every two weeks), I knew with each day after that I would gain strength and feel better than I had in months. A great thing to look forward to.

Of course, close on the heels of that was the second, more vanity-oriented question: How long will it be before I have hair again? Eric and I did a little research, and discovered that the average time it takes for your hair to start growing again is four weeks. I thought "Yay, only a month!" What I didn't think about is that it would take some additional time for the growing hair to get from my hair follicles to my skin. It took about six weeks, but one day I looked in the mirror, and the light was just right, and I could see baby eyebrows starting. I was thrilled, and waving my hand at the mirror said, "Hi, little eyebrows. Welcome back!" It was another week or so before I could feel peach fuzz on my head, but it was a start. I could tell, though, that it would be some time before I could go out without a turban, unless I wanted to sport the bald look.

<u>INSIGHT</u>
So it may seem silly that I talked to my eyebrows, but throughout this entire experience I have talked to my body parts. After a good workout I compliment my various successes: "Good balancing job, left ankle!" After my surgeries I praised my skin and muscles for

---

As the weeks went by, I could feel myself getting stronger every day. Of course I continued my regimen of exercise, meditation and guided imagery, as well as sound healing therapy sessions and Reiki, when my budget permitted. My workouts improved and my interests expanded. I hadn't realized until afterwards how little I had been doing. Chores had piled up on my desk for months. I had barely read any books or played any music. It was such a joy to have my energy improving and my enthusiasm for doing things coming back that the hair was not as much of an issue as I had thought it would be. I had gotten used to the turbans. On the other hand, I do have a journal entry that says "Waiting for hair, waiting for hair, waiting for hair."

About a month after chemo was done I met with the radiation oncologist. They were recommending radiation as a follow up, and I really didn't want to do it. I thought, "Can I be done, please? Didn't the chemo get it all, for Pete's sake? Do I have to have yet *another* insult to my body?" It was depressing. I felt like I was running out of *Julie valiantly and quirkily faces her new challenges* energy. And who wouldn't be, at this point?

But after a few days, I reminded myself again that I didn't have to do what the doctors recommended. That may seem pretty obvious, but the culture of allopathic medicine encourages this kind of thinking: You go to the "wise" doctor, and he or she pronounces the verdict, and you're supposed to dutifully follow their recommendations, because they know best. But they don't always. I can't have lived with Eric for all these years and not know that. I truly appreciate the fact that these people – my oncologist and radiation oncologist for example – do a very specialized thing. It is a rare skill to be able to design and monitor a chemotherapy regimen and not kill the patient. They know what the recommended treatments are and why. They know statistically what treatment plans have the best outcomes. But they often don't know much *outside* their area of expertise. When I suggest straying from the path, they act like I'm being a bad little girl. Eric reminds me "It's all a numbers game. In the end *you* are the most important variable in the equation."

MESSAGE 3: (Reminder) Remember that you are in control of your choices. You have to live with the consequences, but *you* are in charge.

When I went to see the radiation oncologist a second time, she convinced me that statistically my chances of recurrence would be less if I did it. Not a staggering difference, but enough to make it worthwhile. Eric pointed out that the potential side effects from radiation paled in comparison to chemotherapy, which made me feel better, so I agreed to do it. I did rant in the car on the way home. "Damn it! Couldn't I at least have hair before the next scary phase?" And it *was* a creepy thought: Six weeks of getting radiation treatments five days a week. I've spent my whole life trying to avoid excessive radiation. I put off my dental X-rays for as long as I can, and freak out whenever I have to have something big, like a chest X-ray. And here I was, agreeing to do it thirty times in a row.

But once I had agreed to do it, I was determined to not let this last thing get me down. After all, it was the *last thing*.

RULE #14
Never let go of your determination. It can save you.

Before you get radiation they have to "map" you with a

CAT scan, so they'll be sure to aim the machine at the perfect spots. Of course, no one described the procedure to me in advance, so I didn't know exactly what to expect. They just said "We have to send you to be mapped."

So I went in, and the technicians were very nice but they didn't tell me much about the procedure either. They had me lie down, and told me I wasn't allowed to move or talk during the mapping: I was to remain perfectly still. Then they left the room and sat in a little booth that shielded them. Of course, I was really nervous, and the fact that they had to leave the room did nothing to decrease my nervousness. The machine made a bunch a loud, weird noises, and all these beams of different colored light shot at me from different directions. The part of me that freaks out at the unknown thought, "Are those laser beams? Will they hurt my eyes if I look at them? Why doesn't anyone *tell* patients anything?" Once again, I was encountering a situation where the technicians are so used to the procedure that they don't explain everything to the patient. *They* know it's safe, and they sometimes forget that all these things can be scary when they're new to you.

The one saving grace was that I had had the good sense to bring my favorite singing bowls CD with me – I'd learned to always take it along, just in case – and I asked them to play it during the scan. And although I just complained about their insensitivity, at least they had the facilities to play the CD. I've discovered that's pretty universal now. You just have to bring your own stuff. I wonder if they had an option to plug in a smart phone or iPod. Technology is changing so quickly. Anyway, the CD helped immensely, although it was a little weird because they had to turn it up super loud because the machine was so noisy. Still, if the CD hadn't been playing I probably would've jumped off the table and run away.

They also failed to warn me that they were going to tattoo four blue dots on the corners of the area to be treated. That really annoyed me. I mean, not that I had a choice once I had chosen to do the radiation, but being told by strangers that they're going to give you permanent tattoos while you're lying on a table feeling vulnerable was just one more example of how insensitively patients can be treated in mainstream medicine. Those CAT scan technicians put blue dots on people every day, so it's no big deal to them. (And just to add to the insult, it turned out later that my insurance company wouldn't cover their removal, because it was "cosmetic.")

The place where I actually got the radiation treatments was in a different part of the building, and in contrast to the mapping experience, those technicians couldn't have been more sensitive. They even said, "We know this is scary for people, so we try to make it as relaxing and comfortable as possible." And they did. The first day, instead of radiation, you come in for a "trial treatment." They do more mapping and program the machine just for you. They help you to plan exactly how you're going to lie on the table, so that you'll do it the same way every time. Once you're mapped, they stick little stickers on you that the machine reads. It was extremely calming to know exactly how I would be lying, how long it would take, and what the machine looked like. Plus, once again, they told me I could bring CDs and play them during the procedure.

The radiation machine is a magnificent, stunningly huge apparatus. I was simultaneously in awe of the technology and expertise it took to create something that sophisticated and precise, and at the same time terrified of it. It reminded me of torture machines in the science fiction movies I'm so fond of.

The day after the trial run I started my treatments. I wasn't so much freaked out by the idea of the potential side effects; it was the idea of placidly lying there while a big machine zapped me with radiation. I would be nervous and feel like jumping off the table again. So I was nervous about being nervous. Silly, but quite normal.

But I knew if I did the right things, I could overcome

my fear and apprehension, so this is what I did: One, I mentioned earlier how calming humming can be, (see Rule #7) so I hummed during my treatments. I actually had asked my radiation oncologist if I could hum, and she had said no. I assumed that was because she figured it would cause me to move too much, and I was supposed to stay absolutely still. But I had to breathe, of course, so I just hummed on the exhale. *Very* carefully and gently. It helped immensely. It calmed me and distracted me at the same time.

Two: Eric said to me, "Imagine that it's only a couple of particles and it's a tiny stream of radiation. You don't really know how much they're giving you." I realized I had been envisioning being bombarded continuously with lots of nasty beams, and I didn't have a clue what was really going to happen. It reminded me that some of the scary part was in my mind. So I visualized small, weak streams of particles. That was silly, too, but it sure helped.

Three: I decided to go in with a smile on my face and a cheerful posture. Why? Here is a direct quote from another book I wrote called *Keys to Life: Life's Lessons Learned at the Piano*: "Our posture and the expressions on our faces are directly related to how we feel. When we feel lazy or depressed, our shoulders droop, our heads hang, and our faces reflect these feelings as well. While most of us are aware that the way we feel affects both the way we carry ourselves and the expressions on our faces, most people don't realize something really amazing: *the way we carry ourselves and what expressions we put on our faces can change the way we feel.* It works in the other direction, too. We can influence the way we feel by changing our posture and expression."

As it turns out, I am not the first person to notice this, but a lot of people aren't aware of the research on it. A series of studies have been done by Paul Ekman regarding facial expressions and their effect on mood. Anthony Robbins, too, in his wonderful book *Unlimited Power*, devotes a whole chapter to what he refers to as "physiology," and how to change your mood by changing your posture."

So when I walked into the radiation treatment room, I would put a happy and self-confident expression on my face, and carry myself like I was cheerful. And it helped! Not spectacularly, but a little, and every little bit helped.

Four: I remembered one of the affirmation CDs I listened to contained the phrase "I thank this medicine and these proceedings for helping me to become well." That helped me to put a positive spin on it.

Five: I had asked my radiation oncologist why radiation does more damage to the cancer cells than to the "good" cells. She explained that while cancer cells are very aggressive and can multiple quickly, they are weak in other ways, and the radiation harms them in a way that is more deadly to them than the other cells. So I visualized the wimpy cancer cells shriveling and dying (Ahhiiieee…) and my strong other cells bouncing back quickly.

These five things, plus the meditation CD playing in the background were enough to keep me calm and relaxed on the table. It's a good thing I was. The machine was super noisy, and I could tell when it was shooting the radiation because it made a different noise each time it did, which was really creepy.

After a week or so, I came up with yet another strategy. I imagined that I was a crow, flying up and off the table, out the door, and back to my house. I envisioned myself soaring above the buildings and away from anything negative or distressing. That was really fun, actually. And after a week of doing that, I realized with some amusement that I had been flying down the road like I was a human driving a car. I was a crow, after all: I could fly over the treetops and avoid the road. That made my journey all the more spectacular.

RULE #15
If you're going to be a crow, *think* like a crow.

I had been told that radiation therapy can make you very tired, and after about two weeks, I did begin to feel a little fatigued. Not very much, just a little, and I barely noticed it, for which I was grateful. I had started radiation two months after I was done with chemo, and I had been increasing the intensity of my workouts, along with continuing my other habits. I am sure that helped. I also wondered how much of the fatigue was due to the radiation and how much was due to the fact that I was getting up earlier than usual every morning and running over to the hospital for a treatment *before* work. I've never been very good at getting up early. I'm sure, too, that the response differs from patient to patient: where the radiation is aimed, how much, how well they were doing when the treatments started, etc. I was just happy that it wasn't bothering me very much.

<u>CURIOSITY</u>
During my treatments, my hair grew in more and more. I had been waiting for hair, but I wasn't prepared for the fact that *every single hair follicle* started growing at the same time! At any given time, not all of our follicles are active: some hairs grow, others fall out and begin again. There's a cycle to each follicle. But all my hairs had been dormant, and so as the effects of the chemotherapy wore off, they *all* started to grow. This was very nice for the top of my head; as my hair has thinned as I've gotten older, so it looked wonderful. On the other hand, my nose hairs were wild and unruly, and all the little fine hairs on my neck (that you usually hardly notice) were all growing at the same time. It was practically a beard!
Over time, the follicles settled down to a regular routine, but it was certainly an unexpected experience.

So the six weeks of treatment mostly passed uneventfully. Toward the end, however, my skin at the treatment area started to look red and burned, like a sunburn. It was a little worrisome, but I learned that some people got blisters and sores, and I wondered how much my regular regimen was helping. I'll never know, but I was glad that my skin responded so well.

Finally after six weeks I was done. Done with

everything. It was a wonderful feeling. The only residual treatment was a hormone suppressing drug, but that was all. As you can imagine, I was ecstatic.

At the end of chemotherapy there is a ritual where you are supposed to ring a bell that's hanging on the wall inside the infusion center. When I had finished chemo I rang it, not because I wanted to, but because Eric told me to be a good sport. He said even if I didn't care, the *nurses* like to hear it.

There's also a bell in the radiation treatment center. I didn't want to ring that one either, but I appreciated the idea behind it; the ritualistic catharsis. So on the last day of my treatments I took one of my singing bowls with me and played it in the hall where the bell was. It was the perfect solution for me: I got my cathartic ritual but did it in a way that had meaning for me. Many of the staff had never seen a singing bowl, and they thought it was really cool.

STEP 8: Conclusion

If you are a cancer patient, or even if you're not, the question you may be asking at this point is, "What if you did all this stuff and you die of cancer anyway?"

I've asked myself that question many times. In a way, I'd feel pretty stupid praising all my exercise and alternative therapies and then finding out my cancer has recurred and it was all for nothing. But it *wasn't* for nothing.

First of all, I'm going to die of *something*. There's no getting around that. And the older I get, the less it bothers me. Of course, like everyone, I'm hoping to maximize my time here, and die peacefully in my sleep when I'm old, surrounded by my loving family and friends. Pain free would be nice, too, as would having a good *quality* of life up until the end. Frankly, I think I'm more afraid of pain and the unknown than I am of dying. Albus Dumbledore said "It is the unknown we fear when we look at death and darkness, nothing more." (*Harry Potter and the Half Blood Prince*, pg. 566)

Second and more importantly: All of those things I did throughout my surgeries and my treatments made me feel wonderful. In fact, as I said before, more wonderful than I have felt in years. They helped the *quality* of my life during everything I did and allowed me to continue living my life and doing what I love. I didn't have to take a hiatus from my life to get through treatments. Since my treatments ended, I have kept up with all those things: Regular yoga and exercise, meditation, guided imagery, affirmations, and Reiki and sound healing therapy sessions. I didn't just do those things to fight cancer; I did them to heal my body, my mind and my spirit. It was the cancer that galvanized me to go down that path, and I am still walking it.

Of course, it's easier to be diligent about your workouts and meditation, etc., when you feel like you're actively engaged in a fight, so you'd think that once all my treatments were over I would relax my vigilance. But I haven't. For one thing, they have gotten to be such a habit that it feels weird not to do them. I miss them on the days I don't do anything. It just feels wrong. I remind myself that all these activities not only helped me to get well, they help to *keep* me well. On days when I don't feel much like running (that's the one thing I always have to gear myself up for), I make myself go anyway and chant to myself as I run, "We are mending, we are healing, we are healthy. We are mending, we are healing, we are healthy." It gives me the incentive to keep putting one foot in front of the other.

I can't even say I wish I had never gotten cancer. That may sound surprising, but I am a better person for it in many ways. When I was first diagnosed, I was afraid not just of the cancer, but that it would change me, and change the way people perceived me. And I was right; it did. But not in a negative way, as I had feared, but in a very positive way. It has taken me on a new path. I had to endure some horrible things on that path, but it is a *good* path.

RULE #16
Cancer can be an adventure.

My life is fulfilling, and full of joy and love. I am happier, healthier, and more spiritually balanced than I have ever been. That's about the best I can ask for in this life. So yes, I hope cancer doesn't take me out early, but if it does, I'll know I lived my life exactly the way I thought I should – a sentiment I couldn't have stated ten years ago.

BONUS
I mentioned early on that I had had an interest in and had studied sound healing, as well as Reiki, but I had never felt ready to take the plunge into being a practitioner myself. They still felt a little too un-science-y to me to feel confident about my ability to help others using them. I felt like I needed to read studies about how they work, and scientific proof that was irrefutable. Without those I knew I would feel like an imposter as a practitioner. After my experience, it turns out I was my own "proof." I don't know exactly how all these alternative

Appendix I
Rules and Messages

RULES

#1: There's a positive side to everything.

#2: Humor can be found – and often should be – in the most unlikely places.

#3: No matter what the doctors and nurses recommend, remember that they have their own biases as well. Sort the facts, weigh your options, and choose what is right for you.

#4: Cancer can be liberating.

#5: Face the challenge in front of you, and not the ones in your future. Their time will come.

#6: Keep a journal. It helps to get your thoughts and feelings out, and you can say anything you want to *yourself*.

#7: When you have no other resources, hum.

#8: Sometimes it's important to live in the moment. Sometimes it serves you better to focus on the larger picture.

#9: Don't turn gifts away. It's easy to say "Oh, you don't have to bother," or "I'll be okay." Accept the gifts that people offer you. It means something to you *and* them.

#10: Never assume what people are going to think of you. You're seldom right.

#11: Your body is wise. Listen to it.

#12: Never underestimate the positive effect of feeling like you look your best.

#13: Words are powerful. Be mindful of how you use them.

#14: Never let go of your determination. It can save you.

#15: If you're going to be a crow, *think* like a crow.

#16: Cancer can be an adventure.

MESSAGES

#1: Have someone hold your hand, no matter what.

#2: If you don't have someone close to you who knows something about healthcare, do your own research so you don't feel like you're just blindly following your doctors.

#3: Remember that you are in control of your choices. You have to live with the consequences, but *you* are in charge.

#4: Keep exercising. For your body *and* your mind.

#5: Focus on the positive aspects of your life, peacefulness, and the blessings that you have.

#6: If something works to make you healthier, happier, etc., keep doing it and ignore the eye-rollers.

#7: Have something bigger that eclipses day-to-day worries. For me, being close to nature again was bigger than having cancer.

#8: Journaling can be amazingly therapeutic.

#9: We're all going to die. Be your full self while you are here.

#10: If you have good role models, you have an advantage from the beginning. If you don't have any, seek them out!

#11: Keeping perspective is extremely important. Always try to look at your situation from different angles.

<u>**Appendix II**</u>
<u>**RESOURCES**</u>

BOOKS
Gaynor, Mitchell – *The Healing Power of Sound*
http://www.gaynorwellness.com/
Dr. Gaynor was an oncologist who used singing bowls to great advantage in his practice.

Lipton, Bruce – *The Biology of Belief*
https://www.brucelipton.com/
Dr. Lipton is a molecular biologist and an internationally recognized leader in bridging science and spirit. The above book is on epigenetics and how it can relate to mind-body medicine.

Oschman, James – *Energy Medicine: The Scientific Basis*

CDs
Belleruth Naparstak – multiple guided imagery and affirmation CDs, including (but not limited to) reducing stress, healthful sleep, general wellness, and dealing with cancer and chemotherapy. I found them at Amazon.

Deuter
"Nada Himalaya"
"Nada Himalaya 2"
These are my favorite singing bowls CDs, and the ones I found the most relaxing.

OTHER RESOUCES
Weil, Andrew - **www.drweil.com**
Dr. Weil is one of the earliest champions of CAM.

Cash, Alice - **http://healingmusicenterprises.com/**
Dr. Cash devised a set of headphones for listening to music during surgery.

<u>**Appendix III**</u>
<u>**GLOSSARY**</u>

Affirmations – Positive statements designed to counter negative thinking. They can be listened to, repeated, or written down for reinforcement. For an affirmation to be the most effective, it should be present tense, positive, personal and specific. Example: "More and more, I can let go of worrying about things that I cannot control, and focus on my own inner peacefulness."

Allopathic Medicine - An expression commonly used by homeopaths and proponents of other forms of alternative medicine to refer to the broad category of medical practice that is sometimes called Western medicine, biomedicine, evidence-based medicine, or modern medicine. Allopathic medicine uses pharmacologically active agents (such as drugs) and physical interventions (such as surgery) to treat or suppress symptoms of diseases or conditions. Biologist Rupert Sheldrake calls this "mechanistic medicine," because it is based on the principle of seeing the human body as a machine. The expression "allopathic medicine" was coined in 1810 by the creator of homeopathy, Dr. Samuel Hahnemann.

CAM – The common acronym for Complementary and Alternative Medicine. There are many healing systems that fall into this broad category, most of which are not considered part of conventional medicine. This includes – but is not limited to – acupuncture, homeopathy, Chinese medicine, Ayurveda, naturopathy, chiropractic medicine, massage, tai chi, yoga, dietary supplements, herbal medicine, Reiki, Qigong, meditation, biofeedback, dance, art, and music therapies, visualization/guided imagery, and sound healing therapy.

Chanting - speaking or singing words or sounds in a ritualistic way. Chants may range from a simple melody involving a limited set of notes to highly complex musical structures, often including much repetition of musical phrases. Many religious and/or spiritual practices throughout the world make use of chanting as part of their rituals.

Guided Imagery - a program of directed thoughts and suggestions that guide the imagination toward a relaxed, focused state. This can be done using an instructor, recordings, or scripts. Usually the imagery asks the recipient to imagine a peaceful, safe place where he/she can relax and feel very comfortable, such as a garden, a forest, or a beach. Once there the guide unfolds various images. For example, in an imagery about general health and well-being, the recipient might be asked to envision a shining white light pouring down on and entering the body, clearing it of aches, pains and disease, and even clearing the mind of unpleasant or negative thoughts. Guided imagery is based on the concept that the body and mind are connected. By engaging all of the senses, the body responds as though the images are real.

Homeopathic Medicine – A holistic system of treatment that was created in the late eighteenth century by Dr. Samuel Hahnemann (1755–1843). The name homeopathy is derived from two Greek words that mean "like disease." The system is based on the idea that substances that produce symptoms of sickness in healthy people will have a curative effect when given in very dilute quantities to sick people who exhibit those same symptoms. Homeopathic remedies are believed to stimulate the body's own healing processes.

Music Therapy – A system of using music to help with healing, recovery, or cognitive functioning. It is applied in two different ways: active and receptive. In active therapy, the therapist and/or the patient actively participate in creating music with instruments, their voices, or other objects. Receptive therapy is when the therapist plays live or recorded music *to* the patient.

A few examples:

- For patients who are having Physical Therapy to learn to walk again, say after an accident, the therapist will play music with beats at the pace the patient is trying to walk. The patient will entrain to the rhythm of the beat, and the walking becomes easier. This speeds up the retraining process. This type of entrainment has also been used with Parkinson's patients to help them move normally.

- For people who stutter, it turns out they can *sing* without stuttering. The Music Therapist has the patient sing his sentences, and then slowly minimize the singing portion until it's either barely noticeable, or the brain is retrained. For stroke patients who cannot speak properly, the same technique can be used.

- For autistic spectrum children, music is often a way to communicate with them when nothing else will reach them.

- For the elderly, Music Therapy has been used to help them become more alert and active. This usually involves playing them (or having them sing) music from their past. Unlike sound healing therapy, most often Music Therapy involves live or recorded music. In addition, unlike many of these other modalities, Music Therapy is a 4 or 5 year Bachelor's degree, at the end of which you must be certified by the American Music Therapist Association (AMTA)

Psychoneuroimmunology (PNI) - The study of the continuous interaction between the mind, the nervous system, and the immune system.

Reflexology – A therapy based on the principle that there are small and specific areas of the hands and feet that correspond to specific muscle groups or organs of the body. In this system, the nerve endings in the extremities provide a "map" of the rest of the body. Examples are the base of the little toe representing the ear, or the ball of the foot representing the lung. Through the application of pressure on particular areas of the hands or feet, reflexology is said to promote benefits such as the relaxation of tension, improvement of circulation, and support of normalized function in the related area in the body. (Source: **www.drweil.com**)
There is a great video entitled "What is Reflexology" on YouTube at this URL:
https://www.youtube.com/watch?v=z8mWlgKMJZ0

Reiki - A Japanese energy medicine practiced for stress reduction, relaxation, and healing. It is based on the idea that an unseen life force energy flows through all living things and is what causes them to be alive. If one's life force energy is low, then one is more likely to get sick or feel stress, and if it is high, one is more capable of being happy and healthy. The intent of the practitioner is to aid the rebalancing of the energy. Often the practitioner will gently lay his or her hands on the client's body, but some practitioners simply put their hands in the field around the body to assist in the balancing of the energy.

Salt Therapy – In a salt room, a halogenerator grinds up pharmaceutical grade salt into minute particles that become airborne when dispersed into the room. The client sits in the room and inhales the salt particles in the air. It is said to help relieve inflammation and loosen congestion to allow easier and improved breathing, increasing oxygen intake and cleansing the airways of smoke, dust, pollutants and other allergens. (Source: **http://www.saltsoftheearth.com.au**)

Sound Healing Therapy – A type of energy medicine that uses sound and vibration to bring about relaxation and healing. One of the basic tenets of the practice is that certain vibrations can heal if we are exposed to them for a prolonged period; they help to bring our mind, body and spirit back into balance, which is a place of health. This can be done in a variety of ways with a wide range of instruments. One of the most common instruments are the Tibetan/Himalayan singing bowls, but practitioners also use drums, rattles, tuning forks, other types of bowls, crystal pyramids, gongs, singing/chanting, and so on. There is no official certification for it, as it is an alternative practice, so practitioners use a wide variety of terms to describe it: Vibrational Therapy, Sound Healing, Sound Immersion, Singing Bowl Therapy…the list goes on and on. Sound healing therapy seems to be one of the most common and straightforward terms.

Tibetan singing bowls –Traditionally, these are bowls that are used in some Buddhist religious practices to accompany periods of meditation and chanting. More recently, singing bowls have been widely used for music making, meditation and relaxation, and personal spirituality. They have become popular with music therapists, sound healers and yoga practitioners. They are not only used and made in Tibet, however, so they are often referred to as "Himalayan singing bowls," or simply "singing bowls," and can come from Nepal, India, Japan, and a number of other countries.

Toning – The creation of extended vocal sounds on a single vowel and pitch in order to experience the sound and its effects in other parts of the body. There are no melodies, no words, specific rhythms or harmonies - just the sound of the vibrating breath. It is thought that through toning one can immediately experience the effects of sound on physical, mental, emotional, and spiritual well-being. Meditative toning is also thought to help with focusing and relaxation, with releasing negative emotions, and with improving stamina and concentration. (Source: **http://www.lemurianchoir.com**)

<u>About Me</u>

I have worn many hats over the years. I have been playing the piano and performing since I was three and almost too short the reach the keys of my family's piano. I teach college classes in music and individual lessons in piano, voice and guitar. I have released four CDs of original music, mostly singer/songwriter style.

I am also now a sound healing and ReikiSound™ practitioner and instructor, and I facilitate group sound meditations regularly.

I love to write, but mostly write I write when I have something specific that I feel needs to be said.

Other books:
Keys to Life: Life's Lessons Learned at the Piano
Bird Days, a book of poetry.

Visit my website: **www.juliemoffitt.com**
Visit my Facebook page: **http://www.facebook.com/juliemoffitt9**

Read my blog: **http://musicandmeditations.blogspot.com/**

If you have a comment, suggestion, or story you'd like to share, feel free to email me at **madjulie@verizon.net**